This book explores the history of love and provides guidance on cultivating healthy relationships, as well as a dual focus on examining the historical evolution of romantic relationships. It also explores the psychology of love, as well as practical insights into maintaining healthy relationships, boundaries, and priorities within the contexts of single-parenting and blended families. This book highlights the broad and evolving nature of love and relationships, emphasizing the adaptive strategies required in today's family dynamics.

DEDICATION

I owe a heartfelt thank you to my family and friends. They have provided me with encouragement, strength, motivation and believed in me which was needed to bring my writings to fruition. Their support has been my anchor, and for that, I am internally grateful.

I extend my deepest gratitude to the field of Mental Health. The insights and perspectives I have gained through my professional experiences and the dedicated individuals in this field have been invaluable. To understanding of psychological boundaries and emotional health that I have developed in this vibrant field has profoundly shaped the discussions in this book.

I am especially thankful to my colleagues and mentors and mental health Who provided guidance and support as I explored the complex interactions between mental health and relational dynamics. Their expertise helps illuminate the pathways through which healthy relationships can be fostered.

To my readers, thank you for embarking on this journey with me. It is my hope that the reflections and strategies outline in this book will Empower you to cultivate more fulfilling and respectful relationships in your own lives.

Love, in its myriad forms, has perennially been at the heart of human existence, shaping our experiences, relationships, and even our survival as a species. It is a complex, multifaceted emotion, often celebrated as the highest virtue in countless cultures and religions around the world. Despite its universal recognition, the true essence of love remains a topic of much debate and introspection, evading a singular definition. This chapter seeks to explore the vast landscape of love, tracing its historical lineage, dissecting its psychological underpinnings, and examining its cultural expressions. By delving into philosophical discussions and the practical manifestations of love in our daily lives, we aim to provide a comprehensive overview of what love is, how it has evolved, and its impact on human civilization.

Our journey through the concept of love will take us from ancient times to the modern digital age, highlighting how love's core principles have endured even as its expressions and interpretations have transformed. We will uncover the theories that attempt to categorize and explain love, the challenges it presents in various relationships, and the future of love in an increasingly connected yet fragmented world. As we embark on this exploration, it's crucial to acknowledge that love, in its essence, transcends language and definition. It is an experience, a feeling, and a guiding force that is both universal and deeply personal. Through this chapter, we aspire to capture the many dimensions of love, offering insights into its profound mystery and its enduring power to connect us all.

The quest to define love and the pursuit of healthy relationships are as old as humanity itself. Love, a complex amalgam of emotions, actions, and philosophical ponderings, remains at the core of our most profound connections and experiences. It shapes our stories, drives our passions, and binds us in a web of social and personal relationships. In this chapter, we embark on an exploration of love's essence and delve into the dynamics of cultivating healthy, fulfilling relationships. We start by tracing love's historical perspectives, uncovering how our ancestors viewed and valued this powerful emotion. From ancient philosophies to modern psychological theories, we examine the evolution of love and its significance across diverse cultures and times. This journey not only highlights the universality of love but also highlights its diverse expressions and interpretations. Understanding love's psychology provides us with insights into the emotional and cognitive processes that underpin our relationships. We explore how love is woven into the fabric of our mental and emotional wellbeing, influencing our actions and decisions in the pursuit of connection and intimacy.

Cultural contexts shape our expectations and expressions of love, offering a rich tapestry of norms, rituals, and beliefs about forming and sustaining relationships. By examining love through a cultural lens, we gain appreciation for the varied ways love is celebrated and nurtured around the globe. Philosophical reflections on love challenge us to consider its ethical dimensions and its place in a well-lived life. These musings prompt us to ponder the depth of our connections and the values that guide our relationships. The heart of this chapter lies in unraveling the keys to healthy relationships. Drawing from research and real-life practices, we outline strategies for building communication, trust, and respect. We address the inevitable challenges that arise in love, offering guidance on navigating conflicts, maintaining emotional intimacy, and fostering personal growth within the framework of a partnership.

As we weave through the narratives of love and relationship-building, our aim is not only to understand love's intricate nature but also to empower readers with the knowledge and tools to cultivate lasting, healthy connections. Love, in its many forms, is an art and a science, a feeling and a choice. This chapter invites readers on a journey to discover the essence of love and the pathways to nurturing the relationships that enrich our lives. With the introduction set, we're ready to dive into the rich tapestry of love's history, psychology, cultural expressions, and the practical aspects of building and maintaining healthy relationships.

Historical Perspectives of Love

The journey to understand love begins thousands of years ago, spanning across various civilizations, each contributing its unique insights into the nature of this profound emotion. From the philosophical musings of ancient Greece to the romantic chivalry of medieval Europe, the evolution of love reflects a fascinating tapestry of human thought and social development. In ancient Greece, love was dissected into multiple concepts, each capturing a different aspect of love's complex nature. Eros, often associated with passionate, romantic love, highlighted the physical and emotional intensity of love at first sight. Contrasting Eros, Agape represented selfless, unconditional love, the kind that transcends personal desires and seeks the welfare of others. Philia denoted a deep, affectionate friendship, the love between equals, while Storge described familial love, the natural affection among parents and their children. These distinctions provided a nuanced understanding of love, recognizing its varied manifestations in human relationships. Similarly, ancient Indian texts like the Kama Sutra and philosophical works from China, including Confucian and Taoist teachings, offered insights into love's emotional and ethical dimensions, emphasizing harmony, respect, and moral conduct in relationships. The concept of courtly love emerged in medieval Europe, portraying love as a noble, almost divine force that could inspire knights to perform heroic deeds. Though idealized and often unattainable, courtly love celebrated the emotional and spiritual aspects of love, laying the groundwork for modern romantic ideals. The Renaissance further transformed love, blending the spiritual with the sensual. Poets and playwrights, most notably William Shakespeare, depicted love as a powerful, complex emotion that could lead to both sublime happiness and profound tragedy. This period introduced the notion of romantic love as a central component of marriage, a relatively new concept that began to take hold in society.

The Enlightenment introduced a more rational approach to love, emphasizing compatibility, mutual respect, and the social benefits of marriage. However, it was the Romantic movement that fully embraced love's emotional depth. Romantics idealized love as a transcendent force, capable of overcoming societal constraints and personal limitations. This period celebrated the individual's emotional experience of love, influencing how love is perceived and valued in modern times. Today, love continues to evolve, influenced by social, cultural, and technological changes. The democratization of love, where love is seen as a universal right and value, reflects a more inclusive and diverse understanding of love. Modern psychology and sociology have further enriched our comprehension of love, examining its impact on individual wellbeing and social structures. The historical perspectives on love reveal a fascinating evolution of thought and practice. From the ancients to the modern day, love has been celebrated, analyzed, and debated, reflecting the complexity of human relationships. These perspectives provide a foundation for understanding love's multifaceted nature, offering valuable insights into how love has shaped, and continues to shape, our lives and societies.

Moving forward, we'll delve into The Psychology of Love, a section aimed at unpacking the scientific and psychological understandings of love. This exploration will highlight how love impacts our minds and bodies, influencing our behaviors and relationships.

The Psychology of Love

The quest to comprehend love's essence extends into the realm of psychology, where scientists and researchers seek to unravel the mechanisms behind our deepest emotional connections. From the biochemical reactions that ignite feelings of attraction to the long-term bonds that define enduring partnerships, the psychology of love offers fascinating insights into the human heart and mind. Love's initial rush, often described as being "in love," can be attributed to a potent mix of neurochemicals. Dopamine, serotonin, and oxytocin play pivotal roles in generating euphoria, obsessive thoughts, and strong bonds associated with romantic love. Dopamine, associated with pleasure and reward, creates feelings of excitement and happiness, while oxytocin, known as the "love hormone," fosters bonding and trust. This biochemical cocktail not only fuels romantic attraction but also plays a crucial role in the long-term attachment necessary for sustaining relationships. Several psychological theories attempt to categorize and explain the complex nature of love. Robert Sternberg's Triangular Theory of Love stands out for its comprehensive approach, identifying three components of love: intimacy, passion, and commitment. These elements combine in many ways to form different types of love, from fleeting infatuations to deep, enduring partnerships. This framework helps to understand the dynamic and evolving nature of love in relationships. Attachment theory, another significant psychological perspective, examines the impact of early relationships on our adult romantic lives. It posits that the emotional bonds formed with primary caregivers in infancy influence our expectations and behaviors in adult relationships. Secure, anxious, and avoidant attachment styles affect how individuals approach intimacy, trust, and dependency, shaping the health and longevity of romantic connections.

The interplay between love and mental health is profound. Healthy relationships can provide emotional support, reduce stress, and enhance psychological wellbeing. Conversely, relationship difficulties and loss can lead to emotional distress and mental health challenges. Psychology offers insights into coping strategies and communication skills that can foster resilience and emotional intelligence in relationships, contributing to both individual and relational health. Love not only enriches our lives emotionally but also promotes personal growth. Through relationships, individuals are often challenged to develop empathy, patience, and understanding. Love can motivate personal improvement, inspire creativity, and encourage the pursuit of shared goals and dreams. Psychologists emphasize the importance of maintaining individuality within relationships, allowing love to be a source of inspiration rather than dependency. The psychology of love reveals the complexity and depth of human emotional connections. By understanding the biochemical foundations, psychological theories, and the impact of love on mental health and personal development, we can appreciate the power of love to shape our lives. This knowledge empowers us to build stronger, healthier relationships, enhancing our capacity for love and connection. Having explored the psychological underpinnings of love, the next section will examine Love in Cultural Context, showcasing how love is expressed and experienced across different cultures. This will illuminate the diversity of love's expressions and the universal themes that connect them.

Continuing our exploration, we now turn to Love in Cultural Context, a section dedicated to understanding how love is perceived, expressed, and valued across diverse cultures around the world. This examination will highlight the diversity of love's expressions and the underlying universal themes that connect human experiences of love.

Love in Cultural Context

The expression and understanding of love vary widely across cultures, each offering unique perspectives that enrich the global tapestry of human emotion. From the passionate, expressive love often depicted in Western media to the more subdued, duty-bound expressions of love in some Eastern traditions, cultural contexts shape how love is experienced and shown. Exploring these variations not only broadens our understanding of love but also underscores the universal need for connection and affection that transcends cultural boundaries. In many Western societies, love is often associated with romance, passion, and personal fulfillment. Expressions of love are celebrated publicly, with grand gestures and verbal affirmations considered normative. Conversely, in many Eastern cultures, love is more likely to be expressed through actions rather than words, emphasizing duty, loyalty, and the well-being of the family over individual desires. In Latin American cultures, the concept of amor intertwines with family and community, highlighting the importance of extended familial networks and the collective expression of care and support. Meanwhile, in many African societies, love is deeply embedded in the fabric of community life, with strong emphasis on solidarity, care, and mutual assistance among members. Cultural practices and rituals around love and marriage provide further insight into a society's view on love. For example, in India, arranged marriages still play a significant role, where love is often seen as something that grows and develops after marriage, rooted in compatibility and mutual respect. In contrast, in many Western countries, love is typically the foundation for the decision to marry. Japan offers an interesting case of balancing tradition with modernity, where expressions of love may be subtle and indirect, yet the pursuit of romantic love and companionship is highly valued, as seen in the popularity of dating apps and services.

Literature, poetry, film, and media also reflect and shape cultural narratives about love. From the tragic romance of Shakespeare's Romeo and Juliet to the poetic musings of Persian poet Rumi, the arts have always explored love's depths, complexities, and contradictions. In contemporary times, social media and global connectivity are creating a more homogenized culture of love, blending and blurring traditional distinctions. Despite these cultural differences, certain themes in love are universal. The desire for connection, the experience of joy and pain in love, and the pursuit of relationships that provide meaning and fulfillment are common across humanity. Understanding these cultural nuances in expressing and experiencing love can lead to deeper empathy and appreciation for the diverse ways in which love manifests around the world.

The exploration of love in cultural context reveals a rich diversity of expressions and experiences, shaped by historical, social, and economic factors. Yet, it also highlights the universal nature of love as a fundamental human experience. By embracing both the unique cultural expressions of love and the shared human need for connection and affection, we can foster a more inclusive and compassionate understanding of love in its many forms. With a broader understanding of love's cultural dimensions, we'll next delve into Building Healthy Relationships, providing practical advice and insights for fostering love that is both deep and enduring. This section will merge the insights gained from historical, psychological, and cultural explorations with actionable guidance for nurturing healthy, meaningful connections.

We'll now focus on Building Healthy Relationships, a crucial section that applies the insights from our explorations of love's history, psychology, and cultural expressions. Here, we'll offer practical advice for nurturing love that is not only deep but enduring, drawing on scientific research and real-world examples to provide a guide for developing and maintaining healthy relationships.

Building Healthy Relationships

At the core of a healthy relationship is the understanding that love, in all its forms, requires effort, communication, and commitment. Whether romantic, familial, or platonic, relationships thrive on mutual respect, understanding, and the willingness to grow together. This section outlines key components and practices essential for building and sustaining healthy relationships. Open, honest communication is the foundation of any healthy relationship. It involves not only the ability to express one's feelings and needs but also the willingness to listen and understand those of the other person. Effective communication helps prevent misunderstandings, resolves conflicts, and strengthens the bond between individuals. Regular check-ins and open discussions about each other's needs and expectations can foster a deeper connection and mutual respect. Trust builds over time and is essential for a secure, stable relationship. It's fostered by consistency, reliability, and integrity. Trust involves believing in each other's commitment and having faith in the strength of your bond. Creating a safe space where both individuals feel valued and understood is crucial for a relationship to flourish. Trust also means giving each other the benefit of the doubt and working together to overcome challenges. Respecting each other's differences, values, and boundaries is vital for a healthy relationship. This includes appreciating each other's unique qualities and contributions to the relationship. Acknowledging and celebrating successes, no matter how small, can reinforce a positive dynamic. Mutual respect also means understanding and honoring each other's limits and being willing to compromise. Aligning key values and goals can strengthen a relationship, providing a common direction and purpose. This does not mean you have to agree on everything, but finding common ground on fundamental beliefs and aspirations can foster unity and partnership. Discussing future plans, personal goals, and values helps ensure that both partners are moving in the same direction and supports individual and collective growth.

While shared interests and activities are important, maintaining individuality is crucial for a healthy relationship. Encouraging each other to pursue personal interests, hobbies, and friendships outside the relationship can enhance personal growth and bring new energy into the relationship. It's essential to support each other's independence and growth, recognizing that each partner is an individual first. Conflict is a natural part of any relationship, but it's how you handle it that matters. Approaching disagreements with a mindset of finding a solution rather than winning an argument can prevent conflicts from escalating. Listening to understand, expressing feelings without blame, and working together to find mutually satisfactory solutions are key strategies for constructive conflict resolution. Intimacy is not just about physical closeness but also emotional and intellectual connection. Regularly spending quality time together, sharing personal thoughts and feelings, and engaging in meaningful activities can deepen intimacy. Physical affection, according to each partner's comfort level, also plays a significant role in maintaining a close bond. Building and maintaining a healthy relationship is an ongoing journey that requires patience, effort, and commitment from all parties involved. By fostering communication, trust, respect, and intimacy, and by navigating challenges constructively, relationships can grow stronger and more fulfilling over time. The essence of love, in its many forms, thrives in environments where individuals feel valued, understood, and connected. Having provided a foundation for building healthy relationships, we can next explore Challenges and Resolutions in Love, focusing on common issues that arise in relationships and offering strategies for overcoming them. This closing section will ensure the chapter provides a comprehensive guide to not only understanding love but also living it in the healthiest ways possible.

Continuing our comprehensive exploration of love, we now address Challenges and Resolutions in Love, a critical section aimed at navigating the inevitable difficulties that arise in relationships. Here, we'll delve into common challenges couples face and provide strategies for resolving conflicts, enhancing communication, and reinforcing the bond shared between partners.

Challenges and Resolutions in Love

Even the healthiest relationships encounter challenges. Recognizing common obstacles and understanding how to navigate them can help partners maintain a strong, loving connection. This section explores several key challenges and offers practical resolutions to foster resilience and growth in love.

Overcoming Communication Barriers

Challenge: Communication breakdowns can lead to misunderstandings, resentment, and conflict. Whether it's failing to express needs clearly or not listening effectively, these barriers can erode the foundation of trust and intimacy.

Resolution: Cultivate active listening skills, where each partner fully focuses on the other's words without formulating a response or judgment. Express your thoughts and feelings openly and respectfully, using "I" statements to convey your experiences without blaming. Establish regular check-ins to discuss your relationship, ensuring both partners feel heard and valued.

Balancing Independence and Togetherness

Challenge: Finding the right balance between spending time together and pursuing individual interests can be difficult. Too much independence can lead to disconnection, while too much togetherness can stifle personal growth.

Resolution: Encourage each other to pursue personal hobbies, interests, and friendships outside the relationship. Discuss and respect each other's need for space and together time, finding a balance that meets both partners' needs. Celebrate and support each other's achievements and growth, both individually and as a couple.

Navigating Financial Stress

Challenge: Money issues are a common source of tension in relationships, whether it's due to differing spending habits, income disparities, or financial crises.

Resolution: Openly discuss your financial goals, budgets, and concerns. Create a joint financial plan that addresses both partners' needs and priorities. Seek the assistance of a financial advisor if necessary to navigate complex issues and ensure both partners feel engaged and responsible for their shared financial health.

Maintaining Intimacy and Passion

Challenge: Over time, couples may experience a decline in physical intimacy and emotional connection, leading to feelings of distance or dissatisfaction.

Resolution: Prioritize quality time together, engaging in activities that both partners enjoy and that foster closeness. Communicate openly about desires and needs in the relationship, including sexual intimacy. Consider couples therapy or workshops to explore new ways of connecting and reigniting passion.

Dealing with Conflict and Disagreements

Challenge: Disagreements and conflicts are inevitable, but they can escalate and cause lasting damage if not handled constructively.

Resolution: Approach conflicts with a mindset of finding a resolution that benefits the relationship, rather than aiming to win the argument. Practice empathy, trying to understand your partner's perspective. Learn to apologize and forgive, recognizing that both are essential for healing and moving forward.

Challenges in love are not roadblocks but opportunities for growth and deepening connection. By facing obstacles together, openly communicating, and committing to mutual respect and understanding, couples can navigate the complexities of relationships. Embracing these strategies not only resolves conflicts but also strengthens the foundation of love, ensuring that it endures and flourishes over time. This exploration of challenges and resolutions in love concludes our comprehensive chapter on understanding love and building healthy relationships. We've journeyed through the historical, psychological, and cultural dimensions of love, examined practical approaches to nurturing healthy connections, and provided strategies for overcoming common relationship challenges. By embracing the insights and guidance offered throughout this chapter, individuals and couples alike can cultivate deeper, more meaningful relationships grounded in mutual respect, understanding, and love.

Blended families, where parents bring children from previous relationships into a new union, are becoming increasingly common. Successfully blending these families requires understanding, patience, and a strong commitment from all members to work together as a team. The importance of teamwork in a blended family cannot be overstated; it is the bedrock upon which a harmonious and supportive family dynamic is built. Below, we delve into the significance of fostering teamwork in a blended family and provide strategies to enhance this collaborative spirit.

The Foundation of Teamwork in Blended Families

In a blended family, the initial challenge often lies in establishing trust and security among all members. Trust is the cornerstone of any relationship and is especially crucial in a family dynamic that involves merging diverse backgrounds, personalities, and histories. Working together as a team helps build this trust, as family members learn to rely on and support each other through various challenges and adjustments. Respect and understanding are vital in any family but take on added significance in a blended family. Each member brings their own experiences, values, and expectations into the new family structure. Teamwork encourages open dialogue and empathy, allowing family members to appreciate and respect their differences and find common ground. Open and honest communication is essential for effective teamwork. Blended families should establish regular family meetings where each member can express their thoughts, feelings, and needs without fear of judgment. These meetings foster a sense of inclusivity and belonging, ensuring that all voices are heard and considered in family decisions.

Creating a unified vision for the family can help members align on shared goals and values. Whether it's setting household rules, planning family vacations, or discussing long-term aspirations, having common objectives strengthens the team dynamic and provides a sense of direction for the blended family. Acknowledging and celebrating each member's achievements, as well as milestones achieved together as a family, can significantly boost morale and reinforce the value of teamwork. Celebrations can be as simple as a family dinner to honor a child's academic success or a group outing to commemorate a successful family project. Fostering an environment where family members feel supported and understood is crucial for teamwork. Encourage empathy by discussing feelings, practicing active listening, and showing genuine interest in each other's lives. Support can also be shown through acts of kindness, such as helping with homework or offering encouragement during challenging times.

Shared activities and traditions can strengthen bonds and enhance team spirit within the blended family. Activities should be inclusive, allowing all members to participate and contribute. Whether it's a weekly game night, a cooking project, or a community service activity, shared experiences create memories and foster a sense of unity. The importance of working together as a team in a blended family cannot be underestimated. It lays the foundation for a stable, loving, and supportive family environment where all members feel valued and connected. By building trust, establishing clear communication, setting shared goals, celebrating achievements, and encouraging empathy and support, blended families can navigate the complexities of their unique family dynamics and thrive together as a cohesive team.

Teamwork in a blended family not only addresses the immediate challenges of blending different lives but also sets the stage for long-term happiness and fulfillment for all family members. Through collaboration, understanding, and mutual respect, blended families can create a nurturing and harmonious home where every member feels like an integral part of the team.

Single parenting is a journey filled with unique challenges and rewards, requiring a delicate balance of care, resilience, and self-reliance. Entering the dating world as a single parent adds another layer of complexity, blending the pursuit of personal happiness with the well-being of one's child or children. However, finding love and building a healthy relationship as a single parent is entirely possible. This essay explores the dynamics of single parenting and dating, offering insights and strategies for navigating these waters to cultivate a fulfilling, loving partnership that respects the needs of both the parent and child.

Embracing Single Parenthood

Single parents often grapple with the dual role of being the primary caregiver and provider, which can be both empowering and exhausting. Embracing this role fully means acknowledging the challenges without letting them define your entire existence. It involves celebrating the strengths and successes that come from single parenting, such as developing a deep bond with your children and cultivating a sense of independence and resilience. Recognizing these achievements sets a foundation of confidence and self-worth, essential qualities for anyone looking to enter a new romantic relationship.

Deciding to date as a single parent involves more than personal readiness. It also requires considering the well-being and feelings of your children. It's crucial to ensure that you're not just emotionally prepared to open your heart to someone new but also that your family dynamic can accommodate this change. A healthy approach includes reflecting on your motivations for dating, setting clear expectations for yourself and potential partners, and maintaining open lines of communication with your children, appropriate to their age and maturity level.

The journey to finding love as a single parent often involves patience, transparency, and selectivity. Online dating platforms can be a valuable tool, offering the ability to specify your status as a single parent and to search for partners who are open to dating someone with children. When embarking on new relationships, honesty about your parenting commitments and expectations from a partner is key. This openness ensures that potential partners understand and respect your primary role as a parent, setting the stage for a relationship built on mutual respect and understanding. In any relationship, but especially for single parents, setting clear boundaries and priorities is essential. Your children's needs and well-being should remain at the forefront, and any new partner should respect this hierarchy. Establishing these boundaries early on can prevent misunderstandings and ensure that the relationship grows in a way that complements your family dynamic. Introducing a new partner to your children is a significant step that should be approached with care and consideration. Wait until the relationship is serious and stable before making introductions and prepare both your partner and your children for this meeting. Communicate openly with your children about your partner, addressing their questions and concerns with honesty and reassurance.

Communication is the cornerstone of any healthy relationship. For single parents, this means not only communicating effectively with your partner but also with your children. Ensure that your children feel heard and respected throughout the dating process and foster an environment where they can express their feelings freely. Maintaining your independence within a new relationship is crucial. While it's natural to seek support and companionship from a partner, it's important to preserve your sense of self-sufficiency and to continue nurturing your individual relationship with your children. This balance helps prevent over-reliance on a new partner and ensures that the relationship adds to your life without overshadowing your identity as a parent and individual. Support is a two-way street. Just as you deserve a partner who supports you and respects your role as a parent, it's important to be supportive of your partner's needs and boundaries. This mutual support fosters a strong, healthy relationship that can withstand the challenges of blending lives and families.

Finding love as a single parent and building a healthy relationship is a journey marked by self-reflection, patience, and open communication. It requires balancing the needs and well-being of your children with your desires for companionship and love. By setting clear boundaries, maintaining open lines of communication, and gradually integrating your partner into your family life, single parents can cultivate meaningful, loving relationships that enrich the lives of everyone involved. Ultimately, the key to success lies in embracing the complexities of single parenting as strengths rather than obstacles, approaching dating with honesty and openness, and fostering relationships built on mutual respect and support. In doing so, single parents can find not just love but a partnership that enhances their family's happiness and well-being.

In the journey of companionship, where two lives intertwine, the significance of maintaining one's individuality cannot be overstated. This intricate dance of closeness and personal space is foundational to a healthy, thriving relationship. Individuality – the unique set of characteristics, interests, and values that each person brings to a relationship – is as crucial as the mutual affection that binds partners together. Yet, in the warmth of closeness, the lines defining personal space and individuality can sometimes blur, making boundaries an essential element for sustaining both the relationship and the self.

Boundaries serve as the invisible lines that define the scope of how much we intertwine our lives with others. They protect our sense of self, our space, our sanity, and our independence. They are the foundations of respect and freedom within a partnership, allowing each person to remain whole while being part of a union. This chapter delves into the importance of nurturing individuality and setting healthy boundaries, ensuring that each person in a relationship can flourish as an individual and as a partner.

The Concept of Individuality in Relationships

Individuality in relationships is the preservation of one's identity, interests, and personal growth amidst the shared life with a partner. It's about being true to oneself while being in a committed relationship. However, maintaining this individuality poses challenges, such as the tendency to merge identities in a partnership, leading to the potential loss of personal interests and individual growth. Boundaries, ranging from physical to emotional, are essential for defining personal space, comfort levels, and how much sharing is too much. They are pivotal in fostering respect and personal freedom, laying the groundwork for a relationship where both partners feel valued and heard.

This introduction and outline provide a roadmap for discussing the critical balance between individuality and togetherness in relationships, emphasizing the importance of boundaries. As we proceed to elaborate on each section, we will explore the strategies for maintaining one's sense of self, the art of setting and respecting boundaries, and the ways in which individual growth enriches partnerships.

Let us begin with an in-depth exploration of the first detailed section, focusing on the Concept of Individuality in Relationships. This section will highlight the significance of preserving one's unique identity within the dynamics of a romantic partnership and the challenges that may arise in striving to maintain individuality.

Defining Individuality

At its core, individuality refers to the qualities and attributes that make a person unique and distinguishable from others. In the context of a relationship, it encompasses personal interests, values, habits, and the pursuit of individual goals and dreams. Individuality is the essence of our identity—it's what makes us who we are beyond our role as a partner.

Maintaining individuality within a relationship is crucial for several reasons such as.

Personal Growth: It allows each person to continue growing and evolving independently of their partner. This growth enriches both the individual and the relationship, bringing new perspectives and experiences to share.

Emotional Health: Preserving a sense of self is vital for emotional well-being. It helps prevent feelings of resentment or loss of self that can occur when one's identity becomes too entwined with that of their partner.

Relationship Dynamics: An intense sense of individuality contributes to a healthier, more balanced relationship dynamic. It fosters mutual respect and admiration, as partners appreciate each other's uniqueness and independence.

Attraction: Individuality can also sustain and deepen attraction over time. The ongoing process of discovering new aspects of one's partner can keep the relationship vibrant and engaging.

Common Challenges to Maintaining Individuality

Over-Identification with the Relationship: Sometimes, individuals may begin to define themselves solely in terms of their relationship, losing sight of their own interests, friendships, and passions.

Fear of Disconnection: There might be a fear that pursuing individual interests or spending time apart could create emotional distance or disconnection in the relationship.

Guilt and Neglect: Some may feel guilty for focusing on personal growth or interests, perceiving it as neglecting the relationship or their partner's needs.

Lack of Support: A partner's lack of support for individual pursuits can also hinder the maintenance of one's individuality. It's crucial for both partners to encourage each other's personal goals and activities.

Strategies for Preserving Individuality

Set Personal Goals: Continually setting and working towards personal goals helps maintain focus on individual growth and fulfillment.

Cultivate Independent Interests: Engaging in hobbies and interests outside the relationship enriches one's sense of self and brings new energy and perspectives into the partnership.

Maintain Social Connections: Keeping up with friendships and social activities independently of one's partner ensures a support network and a life outside the relationship.

Communicate Needs and Desires: Openly discussing the importance of individuality and personal space with one's partner can help set expectations and build understanding.

The concept of individuality in relationships underscores the delicate balance between being a committed partner and staying true to oneself. By navigating the challenges to maintaining individuality and employing strategies to preserve it, individuals can enhance not only their personal well-being and growth but also the health and vibrancy of their relationships.

Moving forward, the next section, Boundaries: The Foundations of Respect and Freedom, will delve into the types of boundaries crucial for sustaining individuality and the overall well-being of the relationship. Continuing our exploration into maintaining individuality and the importance of boundaries within relationships, we delve into the foundational role that boundaries play. This section examines the several types of boundaries, why they are critical for mutual respect and personal freedom, and how they can be effectively established and communicated in a partnership.

Boundaries: The Foundations of Respect and Freedom

Boundaries in relationships are essential limits we set to protect our well-being and foster a healthy, respectful partnership. These boundaries help delineate where one person ends, and the other begins, ensuring that each individual's needs, feelings, and personal space are acknowledged and valued.

Types of Boundaries

Emotional Boundaries protect your feelings and ensure that your emotional needs are recognized and respected. They involve the right to have your own feelings, free from manipulation or disregard by your partner. Physical Boundaries pertain to your personal space, physical touch, and privacy. Everyone has different comfort levels regarding these aspects, and it's crucial that these preferences are honored. Intellectual Boundaries relate to the respect for ideas and thoughts. Agreeing to disagree is a healthy practice, allowing for individual opinions and beliefs. Time Boundaries ensure that each partner respects the other's time, allowing for personal pursuits, work commitments, and alone time, which are all vital for individual growth. Digital Boundaries have become increasingly significant, involving aspects like social media usage, digital communication, and online privacy. Financial Boundaries involve mutual respect for each partner's financial contributions and decisions, ensuring that financial matters do not become a source of power imbalance or conflict.

The Importance of Boundaries

Boundaries are the underpinning of mutual respect and freedom in a relationship. They allow individuals to

Maintain Individuality: By establishing boundaries, partners can preserve their unique identities within the relationship, preventing the loss of self that can occur in closely intertwined partnerships.

Enhance Relationship Satisfaction: Clear boundaries reduce misunderstandings and conflicts, leading to higher relationship satisfaction. They provide a framework within which both partners can navigate their needs and expectations.

Foster Trust and Security: When boundaries are respected, it builds trust between partners. Knowing that your needs and limits are valued by your partner creates a sense of security and comfort.

Promote Personal Freedom: Boundaries allow for personal freedom, giving each partner the space to grow, pursue their interests, and cultivate their well-being, which in turn enriches the relationship.

Establishing and Communicating Boundaries

Self-Reflection: Identifying your own needs and limits is the first step in establishing boundaries. Understanding what matters to you allows you to communicate these needs clearly to your partner.

Open Communication: Discuss boundaries openly and honestly with your partner. Express why they are important to you and how they contribute to your well-being and the health of the relationship.

Mutual Respect: Boundaries should be established with mutual respect. This means both partners are committed to understanding and honoring each other's limits.

Flexibility: Boundaries may evolve over time as the relationship grows and changes. Being open to revisiting and adjusting boundaries is key to maintaining their relevance and effectiveness.

Establishing and respecting boundaries is crucial for the health and longevity of any relationship. They are the foundations upon which mutual respect and personal freedom rest, allowing each individual to flourish both within and outside the partnership. By effectively communicating and honoring these boundaries, partners can create a balanced, respectful, and fulfilling relationship that nurtures individual growth alongside collective happiness.

As we proceed to the next section, Balancing Togetherness and Individuality, we'll explore practical strategies for maintaining personal interests and friendships, emphasizing the role of personal space and time apart in strengthening the relationship. This part of our discussion will focus on practical strategies that individuals in a relationship can use to maintain their personal interests, friendships, and the crucial role of personal space and time apart, which can significantly strengthen the relationship.

Balancing Togetherness and Individuality

A harmonious relationship is not measured by the quantity of time spent together but by the quality of the connection and the mutual respect for each other's individuality. Balancing togetherness with individuality allows couples to enjoy shared experiences while also nurturing their personal growth and interests. This balance is essential for a healthy, dynamic relationship where both partners feel fulfilled.

Maintaining Personal Interests and Friendships

Cultivating Personal Hobbies: Encourage each other to pursue hobbies and interests outside the relationship. This not only allows for personal growth but also brings new experiences and insights into the relationship, enriching conversations and shared moments.

Supporting Friendships: Maintaining friendships outside the relationship is crucial. These relationships provide additional emotional support, perspectives, and social outlets, contributing to a well-rounded life.

Setting Aside "Me" Time: Regularly scheduled time for oneself—whether for relaxation, contemplation, or pursuing personal projects—helps maintain a healthy sense of self within the relationship framework.

The Role of Personal Space and Time Apart

Fostering Independence: Time spent apart fosters independence and confidence, qualities that are attractive and contribute to a healthier relationship dynamic.

Appreciating Together Time More: Absence can indeed make the heart grow fonder. Time spent apart can lead to an increased appreciation for the moments spent together, making them more meaningful.

Preventing Overdependence: By ensuring that each partner has space to be themselves, relationships can avoid unhealthy patterns of overdependence, which can lead to resentment and a loss of individuality.

Strategies for Achieving Balance

Communicate Needs and Expectations: Openly discuss the importance of individuality and personal space, ensuring that both partners understand and respect each other's needs.

Plan Together Time Thoughtfully: Make the time spent together engaging and meaningful. Quality over quantity ensures that together time is something both partners look forward to.

Support Each Other's Goals and Ambitions: Encourage and support each other in pursuing personal goals and ambitions. Celebrate each other's successes and be there for encouragement during setbacks.

Respect Boundaries: Honor the boundaries each partner sets around personal space and time. Recognize that these boundaries are a sign of a healthy relationship, not a lack of love or commitment.

Balancing togetherness and individuality does require ongoing effort, communication, and mutual respect. By valuing each other's personal space and interests, partners can strengthen their relationship, ensuring that it remains vibrant and fulfilling. This balance allows both individuals to grow and evolve, not just as partners but as individuals, bringing the best of themselves into the relationship.

This section has underscored the significance of nurturing individuality and personal space within the framework of a relationship, highlighting practical strategies for achieving a harmonious balance between togetherness and independence. As we continue to explore the nuances of healthy relationships, focusing next on Communication: Articulating Needs and Boundaries, we'll delve into the essential communication techniques that facilitate understanding and respect for individuality and boundaries within a partnership.

Embarking on the next crucial aspect of maintaining individuality within relationships, we explore Communication: Articulating Needs and Boundaries. Effective communication is the linchpin that holds the complex dynamics of a relationship together, ensuring that both partners feel heard, respected, and valued. This section will delve into techniques for effectively communicating personal needs and boundaries, emphasizing the importance of an ongoing dialogue to foster understanding and mutual respect. Communication: Articulating Needs and Boundaries

Communication in relationships extends beyond mere dialogue; it is about connecting deeply with your partner to share thoughts, feelings, desires, and concerns. It involves listening just as much as speaking, ensuring a two-way exchange that respects and values each partner's individuality.

Techniques for Effective Communication of Boundaries

Use "I" Statements: Frame your communication from your perspective to avoid sounding accusatory. For example, "I feel overwhelmed when I don't have some time to myself during the week" is more effective than "You never give me any space."

Be Clear and Specific: Vague statements can lead to misunderstandings. Be specific about what you need, why you need it, and how it can be achieved. This clarity will help your partner understand and respect your boundaries.

Practice Active Listening: Show your partner that you are engaged and value what they are saying. Active listening involves nodding, making eye contact, and repeating back what you've heard to confirm understanding.

Acknowledge and Validate Feelings: Even when you disagree, acknowledging your partner's feelings fosters a supportive environment. Validation does not mean agreement but shows respect for the other's experiences and emotions.

Timing Matters: Choose the right moment to discuss important matters. A calm, neutral time is more conducive to open dialogue than a stressful or emotionally charged moment.

The Importance of Ongoing Dialogue

Adapt to Changes: As relationships evolve, so do individual needs and boundaries. Regular check-ins can help partners stay aligned with each other's changing needs.

Prevent Resentment: Continuous communication prevents small issues from festering into resentment. Addressing concerns early on maintains the health of the relationship.

Foster Deep Understanding: Ongoing dialogue deepens understanding between partners, making it easier to support each other's individuality and growth.

Cultivate Emotional Intimacy: Sharing thoughts, fears, and dreams openly contributes to emotional intimacy, strengthening the bond between partners.

Challenges in Communicating Needs and Boundaries

Fear of Rejection: Some may fear that expressing their needs or boundaries will lead to conflict or rejection. Overcoming this fear requires trust in the strength of the relationship and the mutual respect between partners.

Miscommunication: Differences in communication styles can lead to misunderstandings. It's important to be patient and willing to clarify and discuss misunderstandings as they arise.

Finding Balance: Balancing individual needs with those of the relationship can be challenging. Open, honest communication is key to finding a compromise that respects both partners' needs.

Articulating needs and boundaries through effective communication is vital for maintaining individuality in relationships. It requires clarity, active listening, and an ongoing commitment to dialogue. By prioritizing communication, partners can ensure that their relationship respects and nurtures the individuality of each person, contributing to a healthier, more balanced partnership. Having explored the pivotal role of communication in articulating needs and boundaries, the journey continues towards understanding how recognizing and respecting each other's boundaries is equally crucial for the health of the relationship. This respect forms the foundation for trust, security, and mutual growth.

Advancing our exploration into maintaining a healthy balance of individuality within relationships, we now turn our focus to Recognizing and Respecting Boundaries. This crucial aspect goes beyond merely setting personal boundaries; it involves both partners actively acknowledging and honoring these limits as an expression of respect and care for one another. Here, we'll delve into how to effectively recognize and respect each other's boundaries and navigate situations where boundaries may be challenged or unintentionally crossed.

In the landscape of a relationship, boundaries serve as essential markers that define each partner's comfort zones, needs, and preferences. Recognizing and respecting these boundaries is fundamental to fostering a healthy, respectful partnership.

Understanding Boundaries

Identify Non-Negotiables: Each person has core boundaries that are non-negotiable. These often relate to personal values, ethics, and deep-seated needs. Understanding and respecting these non-negotiables is key to maintaining harmony.

Learn to Read Signals: Not all boundaries are verbalized. It's important to be attentive to your partner's non-verbal cues—such as body language and emotional responses—that may indicate discomfort or the need for space.

Ask Questions: If you're unsure about what your partner needs or prefers in certain situations, ask. Open-ended questions can encourage your partner to express their boundaries more clearly.

Respecting Boundaries

Actively Listen and Acknowledge: When your partner communicates their boundaries, listen actively. Acknowledge their needs by confirming your understanding and expressing your willingness to respect their limits.

Adjust Behaviors Accordingly: Respecting boundaries may require changes in behavior or compromises. This adjustment is a clear demonstration of your respect for your partner's individuality and comfort.

Support Independence: Encourage and support your partner's pursuits and activities that fall outside the relationship. This independence is vital for personal growth and fulfillment.

Navigating Boundary Violations

Address Violations Immediately If a boundary is crossed, whether intentionally or by accident, it's crucial to address it promptly. Discuss the incident openly, focusing on feelings and seeking understanding rather than assigning blame. Apologize and Make Amends: If you are the one who has crossed a boundary, offer a sincere apology and discuss ways to prevent similar situations in the future. This shows respect for your partner's feelings and a commitment to the relationship's health. Seek Mutual Solutions: Finding a resolution that respects both partners' needs and boundaries can sometimes require negotiation. Approach these discussions with empathy, aiming for solutions that reinforce trust and mutual respect.

Challenges in Respecting Boundaries

Misunderstandings: Misinterpretations of boundaries can lead to conflicts. Clear, compassionate communication is essential for clarifying misunderstandings.

Adjusting to Change: As relationships evolve, so do individual needs and boundaries. Partners must be willing to adapt and renegotiate boundaries as necessary.

Maintaining Balance: Ensuring that boundaries do not become barriers to intimacy can be challenging. It's important to find a balance where individuality and closeness coexist harmoniously.

The mutual recognition and respect of boundaries are crucial for the health and longevity of any relationship. By understanding, acknowledging, and adapting to each other's boundaries, partners can build a foundation of trust, respect, and mutual support. This solid foundation allows both individuals to thrive within the relationship, fostering a partnership that celebrates both togetherness and individuality.

With the exploration of recognizing and respecting boundaries complete, our journey through maintaining individuality in relationships while upholding healthy boundaries draws us next to the final segment, Growing Together as Individuals. This section will highlight how partners can support each other's personal growth, thereby enriching their relationship.

As we proceed to our final segment of this comprehensive exploration, we delve into Growing Together as Individuals. This crucial aspect focuses on the dynamic where partners not only support each other's personal growth and independence but also find that these individual journeys contribute significantly to the richness and depth of their relationship. Here, we explore strategies for encouraging and celebrating individual development, which, in turn, nurtures a more profound and fulfilling partnership.

Growing Together as Individuals

A paradox that many thriving relationships embody is the ability to grow together by growing individually. This growth mindset ensures that each partner can pursue personal ambitions and self-discovery, which enriches their shared life and deepens their connection.

Support Each Other's Goals: Be your partner's cheerleader for their personal and professional goals. Show interest in their projects, offer encouragement during challenges, and celebrate their achievements.

Provide Space for Exploration: Encourage your partner to explore new interests, hobbies, and friendships. This exploration is vital for personal development and brings new energy and insights into the relationship.

Embrace Change: As individuals grow, they change. Embrace and support these changes in your partner, viewing them as opportunities for renewal and deepening understanding within the relationship.

Nurturing Independence

Respect for Autonomy: Acknowledge and respect each other's need for autonomy. Autonomy supports self-esteem and self-efficacy, which are crucial for individual and relational health.

Foster a Sense of Security: A secure relationship environment where each partner feels safe to explore and grow is foundational. This security is built on trust, open communication, and mutual respect.

Individual Time: Encourage and respect the need for individual time apart from the relationship. This time allows for personal reflection, relaxation, and pursuit of individual interests.

Celebrating Individual Development

Acknowledge Growth: Regularly acknowledge and celebrate each other's growth and achievements. This recognition reinforces the value of personal development within the relationship.

Learn from Each Other: Be open to learning from each other's experiences and growth. Sharing insights and lessons can be mutually enriching and can inspire further personal development.

Adapt and Grow Together: Use the insights and changes from individual growth to inspire joint goals, dreams, and projects. Growing individually does not mean growing apart; it can lead to finding new common ground and deeper compatibility.

Challenges and Resolutions

Balancing Together and Apart: Finding the right balance between individuality and togetherness can be challenging. Open communication and regular check-ins can help navigate this balance.

Dealing with Different Growth Rates: Partners may grow at different rates or in different directions. Maintaining open dialogue, empathy, and support is crucial in navigating these differences constructively.

Fear of Change: Growth can sometimes trigger fears of change or loss. Addressing these fears openly and reassuring each other of the commitment to the relationship can mitigate concerns.

Growing together as individuals within a relationship offers a pathway to a fulfilling and dynamic partnership. By supporting each other's personal growth, respecting individual autonomy, and celebrating each person's development, couples can deepen their bond and enhance their shared life. This approach not only enriches each partner's life individually but also contributes to a stronger, more resilient relationship.

This exploration of maintaining individuality within relationships, through effective communication, boundary setting, and mutual support for personal growth, provides a roadmap for nurturing healthy, fulfilling partnerships. Each segment has emphasized the importance of balancing individuality with togetherness, ensuring that both partners thrive individually and as a couple.

This chapter focuses on the importance of going out on dates and generating date ideas requires a structured approach to effectively cover both the rationale behind maintaining a culture of dating within relationships and the creative suggestions for dates. This chapter will explore why dating is crucial for couples at any stage of their relationship and offer a diverse range of date ideas to suit different interests, occasions, and budgets.

Dating in Relationships

Dating, traditionally seen as a precursor to a committed relationship, holds equal importance for couples in long-term relationships. Regularly going out on dates offers a myriad of benefits, from deepening emotional connections to injecting novelty and excitement into the partnership. This chapter aims to underscore the value of maintaining a culture of dating within relationships, exploring both the why and the how of keeping the spark alive through continuous, intentional dates.

Dates provide a unique opportunity for couples to step away from the mundane aspects of daily life and focus solely on each other. This dedicated time fosters intimacy, allowing partners to reconnect, share experiences, and communicate more deeply. Incorporating new and varied experiences through dates keeps the relationship exciting and dynamic. This novelty stimulates the brain's reward system, reinforcing attraction and bonding. Dates offer an ideal setting for meaningful conversations, helping partners understand each other's evolving thoughts, feelings, and aspirations. Regular dates act as a stress reliever, offering a break from routine responsibilities and allowing couples to enjoy each other's company in a relaxed setting. Addressing common barriers to regular dating, such as time constraints, budget limitations, and family commitments, is crucial. This section provides practical solutions and emphasizes the importance of prioritizing the relationship amidst life's demands.

This extensive section provides a wide array of date ideas, categorized to cater to different interests and situations. From adventure-filled outings to cozy at-home dates, the suggestions aim to inspire couples to explore new experiences together, fostering growth, laughter, and deeper connections.

The process of planning dates can be as enriching as the dates themselves. This anticipation builds excitement and adds a layer of joy to the relationship dynamic. Balancing planned dates with spontaneous outings ensures a variety of experiences that can cater to both partners' needs and preferences. Going out on dates is more than a mere romantic gesture; it's a fundamental practice that nourishes the relationship, ensuring it remains vibrant, connected, and fulfilling. This chapter emphasizes the importance of investing time and effort into planning and enjoying dates, highlighting the endless possibilities for growth, discovery, and joy within the journey of love. Given the constraints of our interaction and the depth of the topic, I'll provide a synthesized exploration focusing on key highlights from each section. This approach will give us a well-rounded view of the importance of going out on dates, overcoming common obstacles, and a diverse collection of date ideas designed to strengthen relationships.

The Importance of Going Out on Dates

Strengthening Emotional Connection: Dates are a special opportunity for couples to step out of their daily routines and focus on each other. This quality time is essential for nurturing the emotional bond and intimacy that are the bedrock of a strong relationship. Maintaining Excitement and Novelty: Novel experiences are crucial for keeping the relationship vibrant. Engaging in new activities together can reignite feelings of excitement and attraction, reminding couples why they fell in love. Communication and Understanding: Dates offer a relaxed environment conducive to open and honest communication. Discussing hopes, dreams, and even everyday concerns can enhance mutual understanding and support. Stress Relief and Enjoyment: In the hustle and bustle of life, dates serve as a valuable pause, a moment of relaxation and pure enjoyment in each other's company, which is vital for mental and emotional well-being.

Overcoming Obstacles to Dating

Time Constraints: Scheduling regular date nights can be challenging, especially for busy couples. The key is to prioritize and plan—consider setting a recurring date night to ensure it's a fixed part of your routine.

Budget Considerations: Dates don't have to be expensive to be meaningful. Focus on the experience and the quality time spent together rather than the cost. Many memorable dates are low-cost or even free.

Lack of Ideas: Keeping dates interesting requires creativity. Rotating who plans the date or keeping a "date idea jar" can keep things fresh and exciting.

Children and Family Commitments: For those with children, finding time for dates might require additional planning, such as arranging for a babysitter or scheduling dates at home after the children are asleep.

Date Ideas to Strengthen Your Relationship

Adventure Dates: Try something new and exhilarating together, like rock climbing, kayaking, or attending a dance class. Shared adrenaline-boosting activities can strengthen your bond.

Cultural Exploration Dates: Visit a museum, attend a theater performance, or explore a new cultural festival together. These experiences can add depth and conversation to your relationship.

Nature and Outdoors Dates: Spend time in nature hiking, picnicking, or stargazing. These activities can foster a sense of peace and connection to the world around you.

At-Home Date Nights: Cook a new recipe together, have a movie marathon, or create art together. Home dates can be deeply personal and relaxing.

Educational and Skill-Building Dates: Take a class together, whether it's for cooking, photography, or learning a new language. Growing in knowledge together can be incredibly bonding.

Relaxation and Wellness Dates: Attend a yoga class together, enjoy a spa day, or simply meditate together. Prioritizing wellness together can enhance your emotional connection.

Planning and Anticipating Dates

The excitement of planning and looking forward to dates can be almost as enriching as the dates themselves. Balancing spontaneity with planned outings ensures a variety of experiences, keeping the relationship dynamic and engaging. Regularly going out on dates is fundamental to nurturing a healthy, vibrant relationship. It offers a way to deepen emotional connections, explore new experiences together, and maintain the excitement and novelty that brought you together. Overcoming obstacles to dating and embracing a variety of date ideas ensures that every couple can find meaningful ways to strengthen their bond, regardless of their circumstances.

The Multifaceted Impact of Healthy Relationships

Emotional Support and Stability: At the heart of a healthy relationship is the unwavering emotional support that partners provide for each other. This support acts as a buffer against the stresses of life, offering comfort, understanding, and a safe haven from the external world. The stability that comes from knowing you have a supportive partner enhances mental health and provides the emotional strength to face challenges.

Physical Health and Longevity: Research consistently shows that individuals in healthy relationships tend to enjoy better physical health and may even live longer. The reasons are multifaceted, encompassing lower rates of chronic diseases, better adherence to medical advice, and a lower risk of mental health issues. The positive behaviors encouraged by a supportive partner—such as eating healthily, exercising, and avoiding risky behaviors—play a crucial role in this aspect.

Personal Growth and Self-Improvement: A hallmark of a healthy relationship is the mutual encouragement of personal growth and self-improvement. Partners who support each other's goals, dreams, and personal development not only contribute to each other's happiness but also foster a dynamic of continuous learning and exploration. This environment of encouragement and motivation is fertile ground for personal transformation and fulfillment.

Enhanced Resilience: Life is unpredictable, filled with difficulties. Healthy relationships equip individuals with enhanced resilience to navigate life's challenges. The shared strength, understanding, and problem-solving capabilities developed within a supportive partnership are invaluable resources during tough times. This resilience is not just about weathering storms but also about emerging from them stronger and more united.

Deepened Sense of Meaning and Purpose: Beyond the tangible benefits, healthy relationships imbue life with a deeper sense of meaning and purpose. The connection and shared experiences with a loved one can transform mundane moments into sources of joy and fulfillment. This sense of purpose is often reflected in shared goals and visions for the future, enriching the partners' lives beyond the confines of the relationship.

The Ripple Effect of Healthy Relationships

The impact of a healthy relationship extends far beyond the individuals directly involved. It creates a ripple effect, influencing families, friendships, and communities. Children raised in environments marked by loving, supportive relationships learn valuable lessons about trust, cooperation, and emotional intelligence. Moreover, the positive dynamics exhibited by healthy partnerships can inspire others in their social circles, promoting a culture of kindness, understanding, and support.

Recognizing the profound benefits of a healthy relationship underscores the importance of consciously investing in its health. This investment might manifest in various forms, such as dedicating time for quality interaction, engaging in open and honest communication, and continuously showing appreciation and respect for one another. Like any significant endeavor, the health of a relationship is contingent upon the effort, care, and intentionality brought into it by both partners.

Final Reflections

In conclusion, the pursuit of a healthy relationship is a journey worth embarking upon, offering immeasurable benefits that touch every aspect of life. As we navigate the complexities of human connections, let us remember that the essence of a fulfilling relationship lies in mutual support, shared growth, and the unyielding commitment to nurture the bond that unites us. By investing in the health of our relationships, we not only enrich our lives but also contribute to a legacy of love, understanding, and compassion that transcends our individual experiences.

Notes